47 Organic Juice Recipes for the Pregnant Mother:

Quickly and Easily Absorb High Quality Ingredients Your Body Needs During Pregnancy

By

Joe Correa CSN

COPYRIGHT

ACKNOWLEDGEMENTS

This book is dedicated to my friends and family that have had mild or serious illnesses so that you may find a solution and make the necessary changes in your life.

47 Organic Juice Recipes for the Pregnant Mother:

Quickly and Easily Absorb High Quality Ingredients Your Body Needs During Pregnancy

By

Joe Correa CSN

CONTENTS

ABOUT THE AUTHOR

After years of Research, I honestly believe in the positive effects that proper nutrition can have over the body and mind. My knowledge and experience has helped me live healthier throughout the years and which I have shared with family and friends. The more you know about eating and drinking healthier, the sooner you will want to change your life and eating habits.

Nutrition is a key part in the process of being healthy and living longer so get started today. The first step is the most important and the most significant.

INTRODUCTION

47 Organic Juice Recipes for the Pregnant Mother: Quickly and Easily Absorb High Quality Ingredients Your Body Needs During Pregnancy

By Joe Correa CSN

The period in which a family is expecting a baby should be filled with lots of positive energy and excitement. However, this is also the time to think about your lifestyle habits and most of all, your diet. Every woman faces the same dilemma: what to eat and how much? Naturally, pregnancy comes with some major hormonal changes that affect your usual eating routine and creates different food cravings that might lead to weight gain and the lack of important nutrients for you and your baby.

Some studies show that pregnant women need more protein, calcium, iron, and folic acid. These nutrients should come from a healthy and well-balanced diet. Your proteins should come from healthy sources like lean meat, fish, poultry, eggs, legumes, and nuts. You have to keep in mind that proteins are "builder nutrients" and are crucial for organ development, especially the brain and heart.

Increased intake of calcium is extremely important to build

a baby's bones and teeth. The lack of calcium can create some serious problems.

Iron is another important nutrient you have to keep in mind when planning your healthy pregnancy diet. This mineral is needed to create enough oxygen for the baby. Lack of iron can lead to anemia and fatigue, as well as the increased risk of infection.

Folic acid, also known as folate, is found in foods in the form of vitamin B. This important nutrient helps prevent different birth defects. However, it can be difficult to get the recommended amounts of folic acid through food alone. For this reason, you will be advised by your doctor to take some dietary supplements before and during pregnancy.

The bottom line is that pregnancy is a beautiful and delicate period in a woman's life. But with some small and well-planned changes, you will be getting all the nutrients you need for a healthy pregnancy.

This book is a collection of pregnancy juice recipes that were created to help you increase the intake of important vitamins and minerals within just a couple of minutes per day. I hope this book will serve as your guide in this unforgettable and precious journey you're about to undertake.

47 ORGANIC JUICE RECIPES FOR THE PREGNANT MOTHER: QUICKLY AND EASILY ABSORB HIGH QUALITY INGREDIENTS YOUR BODY NEEDS DURING PREGNANCY

1.   Apple Blackberry Juice

Ingredients:

2 large apples, cored and sliced

¼ cup of blackberries

1 cup of blueberries

1 tsp of pure mint extract, sugar-free

½ cup of water

Preparation:

Wash the apples and remove the core. Cut into bite-sized pieces and set aside.

Combine blackberries and blueberries in a colander and wash under cold running water. Drain and set aside.

Now, combine apples, blackberries, and blueberries in a

juicer and process until juiced. Transfer to serving glasses and stir in the mint extract and water.

Add few ice cubes before serving.

Enjoy!

Nutritional information per serving: Kcal: 368, Protein: 2.5g, Carbs: 94g, Fats: 1.5g

2.   Basil Celery Juice

Ingredients:

1 cup of fresh basil

1 cup of fresh celery, chopped

2 large tomatoes, chopped

½ tsp of salt

½ tsp of dried oregano, ground

Preparation:

Combine basil and celery in a colander and wash under cold running water. Torn with hands and set aside.

Wash the tomatoes and place them in a bowl. Cut into quarters and reserve the juice while cutting. Set aside.

Now, combine basil, celery, and tomatoes in a juicer and process until juiced.

Transfer to serving glasses and stir in the reserved tomato juice, salt. Sprinkle with some oregano for some extra taste.

Refrigerate for 5 minutes before serving.

Nutrition information per serving: Kcal: 64, Protein: 4.6g, Carbs: 17.8g, Fats: 1.1g

3.   Beet Apple Juice

Ingredients:

1 cup of beets, trimmed

1 large red apple, cored

1 cup of fresh strawberries

1 large lime, peeled

1 ginger root knob, 1-inch

1 tbsp of liquid honey

2 oz of water

Preparation:

Wash the beets and trim off the green parts. Cut into small pieces and fill the measuring cup. Reserve the beet greens for some other juice. Set aside.

Wash the apple and remove the core. Cut into bite-sized pieces. Set aside.

Place the strawberries in a colander and wash under cold running water. Drain and cut in half. Set aside.

Peel the lime and cut lengthwise in half. Set aside.

Peel the ginger root knob and set aside.

Now, combine beets, apple, strawberries, and ginger in a juicer and process until juiced. Transfer to serving glasses and stir in honey and water.

Add some ice and serve immediately.

Nutrition information per serving: Kcal: 277, Protein: 4.2g, Carbs: 82.4g, Fats: 1.3g

4.   Lime Melon Juice

Ingredients:

1 large lime, peeled

2 large honeydew melon wedges

1 cup of fresh mint, torn

1 large yellow apple, cored

2 oz of coconut water

Preparation:

Peel the lime and cut lengthwise in half. Set aside.

Cut the honeydew melon lengthwise in half. Scoop out the seeds using a spoon. Cut two large wedges and peel them. Cut into small chunks and place in a bowl. Wrap the rest of the melon in a plastic foil and refrigerate.

Wash the mint thoroughly under cold running water. Drain and torn with hands. Set aside.

Wash the apple and remove the core. Cut into bite-sized pieces and set aside.

Now, combine lime, honeydew melon, mint, and apple in a juicer. Transfer to serving glasses and stir in the coconut water.

Add some ice and serve immediately.

Nutrition information per serving: Kcal: 228, Protein: 3.4g, Carbs: 65.7g, Fats: 1g

5.   Cabbage Beet Juice

Ingredients:

1 cup of purple cabbage, chopped

1 large beet, trimmed

1 cup of pineapple chunks

1 large carrot, sliced

1 cup of fresh spinach, torn

1 tbsp of liquid honey

Preparation:

Cut the top of a pineapple and peel it using a sharp knife. Cut into small chunks and fill the measuring cup. Reserve the rest of the pineapple in a refrigerator.

Wash the purple cabbage and spinach thoroughly torn with hands. Set aside.

Wash the beet and trim off the green parts. Cut into small pieces and set aside.

Wash the carrot and cut into thick slices. Set aside.

Now, combine cabbage, beet, pineapple, carrot, and spinach in a juicer and process until juiced.

Transfer to serving glasses and stir in the liquid honey. Add few ice cubes and serve immediately.

Enjoy!

Nutrition information per serving: Kcal: 205, Protein: 5g, Carbs: 62.1g, Fats: 0.7g

6.   Swiss Chard Cucumber Juice

Ingredients:

1 cup of fresh parsley, torn

2 cups of Swiss chard, torn

1 large cucumber, sliced

1 small yellow apple, cored

1 small orange, peeled

Preparation:

Combine Swiss chard and parsley in a colander and wash thoroughly under cold running water. Drain and torn with hands. Set aside.

Wash the cucumber and cut into thick slices. Set aside.

Wash the apple and remove the core. Cut into bite-sized pieces and set aside.

Peel the orange and divide into wedges. Set aside.

Now, combine Swiss chard, cucumber, parsley, apple, and orange in a juicer and process until juiced. Transfer to serving glasses and add some ice before serving.

Enjoy!

Nutrition information per serving: Kcal: 161, Protein: 6.3g, Carbs: 46.3g, Fats: 1.2g

7.　　Green Orange Juice

Ingredients:

1 cup of collard greens, chopped

1 cup of Swiss chard, chopped

1 large orange, peeled

1 cup of red leaf lettuce, chopped

1 cup of Romaine lettuce, chopped

1 large cucumber

1 large lemon, peeled

2 oz of water

Preparation:

Combine collard greens, Swiss chard, red leaf lettuce, and Romaine lettuce in a colander. Wash under cold running water and drain. Torn with hands and set aside.

Peel the orange and divide into wedges. Set aside.

Wash the cucumber and cut into thick slices. Set aside.

Peel the lemon and cut lengthwise in half. Set aside.

Now, combine collard greens, Swiss chard, orange, red leaf

lettuce, Romaine lettuce, cucumber, and lemon in a juicer and process until juiced.

Transfer to serving glasses and stir in the water.

Add some ice and serve immediately.

Nutrition information per serving: Kcal: 136, Protein: 7g, Carbs: 43.4g, Fats: 1.2g

8.   Beet Radish Juice

Ingredients:

1 cup of beets, trimmed and chopped

1 large radish, chopped

1 large orange, peeled

1 cup of fresh kale, chopped

1 large cucumber

Preparation:

Wash the beets and trim off the green parts. Chop into bite-sized pieces and set aside.

Wash the radish and trim off the green parts. Cut into small pieces and set aside.

Peel the orange and divide into wedges. Set aside.

Wash the kale thoroughly under cold running water. Drain and torn with hands. Set aside.

Wash the cucumber and cut into thick slices. Set aside.

Now, combine beets, radish, orange, kale, and cucumber in a juicer and process until juiced.

Transfer to serving glasses and add some ice before serving.

Enjoy!

Nutrition information per serving: Kcal: 174, Protein: 8.8g, Carbs: 51.7g, Fats: 1.4g

9.   Tomato Swiss Chard Juice

Ingredients:

1 large tomato, chopped

1 cup of Swiss chard, torn

1 cup of asparagus, trimmed

1 cup of Brussels sprouts, trimmed

1 large cucumbers, sliced

Preparation:

Wash the tomato and place in a bowl. Cut into quarters and reserve the juice while cutting. Set aside.

Wash the Swiss chard thoroughly under cold running water. Drain and set aside.

Wash the asparagus and trim off the woody ends. Cut into 1-inch pieces and set aside.

Wash the Brussels sprouts and trim off the outer layers. Cut in half and set aside.

Wash the cucumber and cut into thick slices. Set aside.

Now, combine tomato, Swiss chard, asparagus, Brussels sprouts, and cucumber in a juicer and process until juiced.

Transfer to serving glasses and add some ice before serving.

Nutrition information per serving: Kcal: 109, Protein: 10.1g, Carbs: 32.4g, Fats: 1.2g

10.   Avocado Cucumber Juice

Ingredients:

1 cup of avocado, chopped

1 large cucumber, sliced

1 large tomato, chopped

1 large lemon, peeled

1 cup of fresh basil, chopped

Preparation:

Peel the avocado and cut in half. Remove the pit and cut into chunks. Fill the measuring cup and reserve the rest for some other juice. Keep it in a refrigerator.

Wash the cucumber and cut into thick slices. Set aside.

Wash the tomato and place in a bowl. Cut into quarters and reserve the juice while cutting. Set aside.

Peel the lemon and cut lengthwise in half. Set aside.

Wash the basil thoroughly and roughly chop it. Set aside.

Now, combine avocado, cucumber, tomato, lemon and basil in a juicer and process until juiced.

Transfer to serving glasses and add some ice before serving.

Enjoy!

Nutrition information per serving: Kcal: 240, Protein: 3.1g, Carbs: 75.1g, Fats: 0.9g

11.   Coconut Squash Juice

Ingredients:

½ cup of coconut water, unsweetened

1 cup of butternut squash, chunked

1 medium-sized banana, peeled

1 cup of raspberries, fresh

1 tsp of honey, raw

Preparation:

Peel the butternut squash and remove the seeds using a spoon. Cut into small cubes and reserve the rest of the squash for some other recipe. Wrap in a plastic foil and refrigerate.

Peel the banana and cut into chunks. Set aside.

Wash the raspberries under cold running water. Drain and set aside.

Now, combine butternut squash, banana, and raspberries in a juicer. Transfer to serving glasses and stir in the coconut water and honey.

Add some ice and serve immediately.

Enjoy!

Nutritional information per serving: Kcal: 197, Protein: 4.7g, Carbs: 68g, Fats: 1.3g

12.   Cranberry Coconut Juice

Ingredients:

1 cup of cranberries

3 oz of coconut water

1 cup of blackberries

1 cup of blueberries

1 cup of strawberries, chopped

1 cup of raspberries

Preparation:

Combine cranberries, blackberries, blueberries, strawberries, and raspberries in a large colander. Rinse well under cold running water. Drain and separate the strawberries.

Cut the strawberries into bite-sized pieces and set aside.

Now, combine all in a juicer and process until juiced. Transfer to serving glasses and add some ice before serving. Optionally, add some honey for some extra taste.

Enjoy!

Nutrition information per serving: Kcal: 210, Protein: 5.9g, Carbs: 75.3g, Fats: 2.5g

13.   Lettuce Orange Juice

Ingredients:

3 cups of red leaf lettuce, torn

1 large orange, peeled

1 cup of avocado, sliced

½ cup of pure coconut water, unsweetened

1 tsp of liquid honey

Preparation:

Wash the lettuce thoroughly under cold running water. Torn with hands and set aside.

Peel the orange and divide into wedges. Set aside.

Peel the avocado and cut in half. Remove the pit and chop into chunks. Fill the measuring cup and reserve the rest for some other juice. Set aside.

Now, combine lettuce, orange, and avocado in a juicer and process until juiced.

Transfer to serving glasses and refrigerate for 5 minutes before serving.

Enjoy!

Nutrition information per serving: Kcal: 240, Protein: 4.9g, Carbs: 25.6g, Fats: 21.7g

14.   Brussels Sprout Carrot Juice

Ingredients:

1 cup of Brussels sprouts, chopped

1 cup of carrots, sliced

1 cup of broccoli, chopped

1 cup of turnip greens, chopped

4 large oranges, peeled

1 tbsp of honey

¼ cup of pure coconut water

Preparation:

Wash the Brussels sprouts and trim off the outer layers. Cut in half and set aside.

Wash the carrots and cut into thin slices. Set aside.

Wash the broccoli and cut into small pieces. Set aside.

Wash the turnip greens thoroughly and torn with hands. Set aside.

Peel the oranges and divide into wedges. Set aside.

Now, combine broccoli, Brussels sprouts, carrots, turnip

greens, and oranges in a juicer and process until juiced. Transfer to serving glasses and stir in the honey and coconut water.

Add some ice cubes before serving or refrigerate for 5 minutes.

Enjoy!

Nutrition information per serving: Kcal: 367, Protein: 14.47g, Carbs: 116g, Fats: 1.9g

15.   Kiwi Spinach Juice

Ingredients:

1 large kiwi, peeled

1 cup of fresh spinach, chopped

5 apricots, sliced

1 large peach, sliced

1 tbsp of fresh mint, chopped

¼ cup of water

Preparation:

Peel the kiwi and cut lengthwise in half. Set aside.

Wash the spinach and mint under cold running water. Drain and roughly chop it. Set aside.

Wash the apricots and cut in half. Remove the pits and cut into chunks. Set aside.

Wash the peach and cut in half. Remove the pit and cut into small pieces. Set aside.

Now, combine kiwi, spinach, apricots, peach, and mint in a juicer and process until juiced.

Transfer to serving glasses and refrigerate before serving.

Nutrition information per serving: Kcal: 211, Protein: 2.8g, Carbs: 58.8g, Fats: 2.8g

16.   Lime Broccoli Juice

Ingredients:

2 whole limes, peeled

2 cups of raw broccoli, chopped

1 cup of fresh raspberries

½ cup of coconut water, unsweetened

2 large cucumbers, peeled and sliced

1 tbsp of honey

Preparation:

Peel the limes and cut lengthwise in half. Set aside.

Wash the broccoli and cut into small pieces. Set aside.

Wash the raspberries under cold running water. Drain and set aside.

Wash the cucumbers and cut into thick slices. Set aside.

Combine limes, broccoli, raspberries, and cucumber in a juicer and process until juiced. Transfer to serving glasses and stir in the coconut water and honey.

Add some ice and serve.

Nutritional information per serving: Kcal: 192, Protein: 10.9g, Carbs: 56g, Fats: 2.2g

17.   Radish Swiss Chard Juice

Ingredients:

1 large radish, chopped

1 cup of Swiss chard, torn

1 large honeydew melon wedge

1 cup of asparagus

1 cup of avocado, chopped

¼ cup of pure coconut water, unsweetened

Preparation:

Wash the radish and trim off the green parts. Cut into small pieces and set aside.

Wash the chard thoroughly and torn with hands. Set aside.

Cut the honeydew melon lengthwise in half. Scoop out the seeds using a spoon. Cut the large wedges and peel them. Cut into small chunks and place in a bowl. Wrap the rest of the melon in a plastic foil and refrigerate.

Wash the asparagus and trim off the woody ends. Chop into small pieces and set aside.

Peel the avocado and cut in half. Remove the pit and cut

into chunks. Set aside.

Now, combine radish, chard, melon, asparagus, and avocado in a juicer and process until juiced.

Transfer to serving glasses and refrigerate 10 minutes before serving.

Nutritional information per serving: Kcal: 275, Protein: 8g, Carbs: 35.2g, Fats: 21,9g

18.   Coconut Guava Juice

Ingredients:

1 large guava, chopped

¼ cup of pure coconut water, unsweetened

1 tbsp of pure coconut sugar

1 small ginger root slice, peeled and chopped

2 cups of Swiss chard, torn

2 cups of fresh kale, torn

A bunch of spinach, torn

Preparation:

Wash the guava and cut into chunks. Set aside.

Peel the ginger slice and set aside.

Combine Swiss chard, kale, and spinach in a colander and wash thoroughly under cold running water. Drain and torn with hands. Set aside.

Now, combine guava, ginger, Swiss chard, kale, and spinach in a juicer and process until juiced.

Transfer to serving glasses and stir in the coconut water

and pure coconut sugar.

Add some ice and serve immediately.

Nutrition information per serving: Kcal: 267, Protein: 22.3g, Carbs: 45g, Fats: 3.8g

19.　　Nutmeg Apple Juice

Ingredients:

1 small apple, peeled and seeds removed

1 cup of pineapple, chunked

1 tsp of fresh mint leaves, finely chopped

¼ tsp of nutmeg, ground

Preparation:

Wash the apple and remove the core. Cut into bite-sized pieces and set aside.

Cut the top of a pineapple and peel it using a sharp knife. Cut into small chunks. Reserve the rest of the pineapple in a refrigerator.

Combine apple and pineapple and process in a juicer. Transfer to a serving glasses and stir in the nutmeg. Add more water to increase the juice amount.

Garnish with mint leaves and refrigerate before serving.

Nutritional information per serving: Kcal: 141, Protein: 1.5g, Carbs: 41.2g, Fats: 0.4g

20.   Blueberry Carrot Juice

Ingredients:

1 cup of fresh blueberries

2 large carrots, sliced

1 small apple, cored and chopped

1 head romaine lettuce, torn

Preparation:

Wash the blueberries under cold running water. Set aside aside.

Wash the carrots and cut into thick slices. Set aside.

Wash the apple and remove the core. Cut into bite-sized pieces and set aside.

Wash the lettuce thoroughly and torn with hands. Set aside.

Now, process blueberries, carrots, apple, and lettuce in a juicer. Transfer to serving glasses and add few ice cubes.

Serve immediately.

Nutritional information per serving: Kcal: 228, Protein: 6.14g, Carbs: 66.8g, Fats: 1.95g

21.   Grape Orange Juice

Ingredients:

½ cup of fresh grapes

3 large oranges, peeled

1 medium-sized pear, roughly chopped

1 cup of spinach, torn

1 small ginger root slice, peeled

Preparation:

Wash the grapes in a colander under cold running water and set aside.

Peel the oranges and divide into wedges. Set aside.

Wash the pear and remove the core. Cut into small pieces and set aside.

Wash the spinach thoroughly and torn with hands. Set aside.

Peel the ginger slice and set aside.

Combine grapes, oranges, pear, spinach, and ginger in a juicer and process until juiced.

Transfer to serving glasses and refrigerate for 10 minutes before serving.

Enjoy!

Nutritional information per serving: Kcal: 347, Protein: 6.52g, Carbs: 108.8g, Fats: 1.27g

22.   Sweet Banana Orange Juice

Ingredients:

1 large banana, peeled

1 large orange, peeled

1 cup of parsnips, sliced

1 cup of cauliflower, chopped

A handful of fresh mint, chopped

1 tsp of honey, raw

Preparation:

Peel the banana and cut into chunks. Set aside.

Peel the orange and divide into wedges. Set aside.

Wash the parsnips and cut into thick slices. Set aside.

Trim off the outer leaves of cauliflower. Wash it and cut into small pieces. Reserve the rest in the refrigerator.

Now, combine banana, orange, parsnips, and cauliflower in a juicer and process until juiced. Transfer to serving glasses and stir in the honey. Sprinkle with mint and refrigerate for 5 minutes before serving.

Enjoy!

Nutritional information per serving: Kcal: 336, Protein: 8.5g, Carbs: 103g, Fats: 1.5g

23.   Coconut Lemon Juice

Ingredients:

½ cup of coconut water, unsweetened

2 large lemons, peeled

1 cup of broccoli, chopped

A bunch of fresh spinach

1 medium-sized orange

1 tbsp of honey, raw

A few mint leaves

Preparation:

Peel the lemons and cut lengthwise in half. Set aside.

Wash the broccoli and trim off the outer leaves. Set aside.

Wash the spinach thoroughly and torn with hands. Set aside.

Peel the orange and divide into wedges. Set aside.

Now, combine broccoli, spinach, lemons, and orange in a juicer and process until juiced. Transfer to serving glasses and stir in the honey and garnish with mint leaves.

Add some ice and serve.

Nutritional information per serving: Kcal: 171, Protein: 14.8g, Carbs: 54.5g, Fats: 2.17g

24. Kale Cranberries Juice

Ingredients:

1 cup of kale, torn

1 cup of cranberries

3 large kiwis, peeled

1 tsp of pure coconut sugar

Preparation:

Wash the kale thoroughly and torn with hands. Set aside.

Wash the cranberries under cold running water. Drain and set aside.

Peel the kiwis and cut lengthwise in half. Set aside.

Now, combine kiwis, kale, and cranberries in a juicer. Transfer to serving glasses and stir in the coconut water.

Add some ice and serve!

Nutritional information per serving: Kcal: 153, Protein: 5.6g, Carbs: 48.4g, Fats: 1.8g

25. Baby Spinach Ginger Juice

Ingredients:

¼ cup of baby spinach

½ tsp of ginger, ground

1 cup of blackberries

1 cup of blueberries

1 cup of raspberries

1 cup of strawberries, chopped

Preparation:

Wash the spinach thoroughly and torn with hands. Set aside.

Combine all berries in a colander and wash under cold running water. Set aside.

Now, mix all berries and spinach in a juicer and process until juiced. Transfer to serving glasses and stir in the ginger.

Add few ice cubes and serve immediately.

Enjoy!

Nutritional information per serving: Kcal: 158, Protein: 5.9g, Carbs: 56.4g, Fats: 2.3g

26.   Grapefruit Honey Juice

Ingredients:

1 large grapefruit, peeled

1 tsp of honey, raw

2 large Granny Smith apples, cored and chopped

½ tsp of ginger, freshly ground

Preparation:

Wash the grapefruit and chop into small pieces. Set aside.

Wash the apples and remove the core. Chop into bite-sized pieces and set aside.

Combine grapefruit and apples and process in a juicer. Transfer to serving glasses and stir in the honey and ginger.

Refrigerate or add some ice and serve.

Enjoy!

Nutritional information per serving: Kcal: 299, Protein: 3.7g, Carbs: 88g, Fats: 1.1g

27.   Spinach Banana Juice

Ingredients:

2 cups of spinach, chopped

1 medium-sized banana, sliced

2 cups of fresh strawberries, chopped

14 oz melon, roughly chopped

½ tsp of cinnamon

1 tsp of honey, raw

Preparation:

Wash the spinach thoroughly and torn with hands. Set aside.

Peel the banana and cut into small chunks. Set aside.

Wash the strawberries under cold running water and chop into small pieces. Set aside.

Cut the melon in half. Cut two large wedges and peel. Cut into small chunks and remove the seeds. Set aside.

Now, combine spinach, banana, strawberries, and melon in a juicer and process until juiced. Transfer to serving glasses and stir in the honey and cinnamon.

Refrigerate for 5 minutes before serving minutes.

Nutritional information per serving: Kcal: 349, Protein: 7.6g, Carbs: 104.9g, Fats: 3.2g

28.   Pineapple Mango Juice

Ingredients:

1 cup of pineapple chopped

1 cup of mango, chopped

½ cup of coconut water

1 cup of guava, chopped

1 tbsp of fresh mint leaves

Preparation:

Cut the top of a pineapple and peel it using a sharp knife. Cut into small pieces. Reserve the rest of the pineapple in a refrigerator.

Peel the mango and cut into small pieces. Set aside.

Wash the guava and cut into pieces. If you are using large fruit, reserve the rest for some other recipe in a refrigerator.

Now, combine pineapple, mango, and guava in a juicer.

Transfer to serving glasses and stir in the coconut water.

Garnish with some mint leaves and add some ice before serving.

Enjoy!

Nutritional information per serving: Kcal: 187, Protein: 3.6g, Carbs: 54.2g, Fats: 1.3g

29.   Blueberry Coconut Juice

Ingredients:

1 cup of blueberries

½ cup of coconut water, unsweetened

2 cups of strawberries, chopped

½ large red orange

1 tsp of pure coconut sugar

Preparation:

Combine blueberries and strawberries in a colander and wash under cold running water. Set aside.

Peel the orange and divide into wedges. Use about half of the wedges and reserve the rest for some other juice.

Combine blueberries, strawberries, and orange in a juicer. Transfer to serving glasses and stir in the coconut water and coconut sugar.

Add some ice or refrigerate before serving.

Nutritional information per serving: Kcal: 246, Protein: 4.7g, Carbs: 74.2g, Fats: 1.7g

30.   Raspberry Blueberry Juice

Ingredients:

2 cups of raspberries

1 cup of blueberries

½ cup of coconut water, unsweetened

½ tsp of pure vanilla extract, sugar-free

¼ tsp of cinnamon, ground

Preparation:

Wash the raspberries and blueberries under cold running water. Drain well. Transfer all to a juicer and process until juiced.

Transfer to serving glasses and stir in the coconut water, vanilla extract, and cinnamon.

Add few ice cubes and serve immediately.

Enjoy!

Nutritional information per serving: Kcal: 136, Protein: 4.4g, Carbs: 51.7g, Fats: 2.4g

31.   Beet Tomato Juice

Ingredients:

1 cup of beets

3 large tomatoes, peeled

2 large apples, cored and peeled

1 cup of goji berries

1 cup of fresh cherries, pitted

Preparation:

Wash the beets and trim off the green parts. Cut into small pieces and set aside.

Place the tomatoes in a bowl and chop into quarters. Reserve the juice while cutting.

Wash the cherries and remove the pits. Set aside.

Wash the apples and remove the core. Cut into bite-sized pieces and set aside.

Place the goji berries in a medium bowl and add 1 cup of water. Soak for 30 minutes before juicing.

Now, combine apples, goji berries, beets, cherries, and tomatoes in a juicer.

Transfer to serving glasses and stir in the reserved tomato juice.

Refrigerate for 10 minutes before serving.

Nutritional information per serving: Kcal: 328, Protein: 9.3g, Carbs: 95g, Fats: 2.14g

32.   Orange Goji Juice

Ingredients:

1 large orange, peeled

1 cup of goji berries

10 oz broccoli, pre-cooked

1 large cucumber, peeled

1 tbsp of honey, raw

Preparation:

Peel the orange and divide into wedges. Set aside.

Place the goji berries in a medium bowl. Add 1 cup of water and soak for 30 minutes.

Wash the broccoli and chop into small pieces. Set aside.

Wash the cucumber and cut into thick slices. Set aside.

Now, process orange, goji berries, broccoli, and cucumber in a juicer. Transfer to serving glasses and stir in the honey.

Add some ice and serve!

Nutritional information per serving: Kcal: 193, Protein: 9.4g, Carbs: 66g, Fats: 1.7g

33.   Banana Honey Juice

Ingredients:

1 large banana, peeled

1 tsp of honey

1 cup of blueberries

1 cup of blackberries

½ tsp of cinnamon

Preparation:

Peel the banana and chop into chunks. Set aside.

Combine blueberries and blackberries in a colander and wash under cold running water. Drain and set aside.

Now, combine banana, blueberries, and blackberries in a juicer and process until juiced.

Transfer to serving glasses and stir in the honey and cinnamon.

Add some ice and serve immediately.

Enjoy!

Nutritional information per serving: Kcal: 229, Protein: 4.5g, Carbs: 76.3g, Fats: 1.6g

34.   Tangerine Coffee Juice

Ingredients:

4 whole tangerines, peeled and wedged

½ cup of chilled coffee

1 tsp of pure vanilla extract

1 tsp of pure coconut sugar

Preparation:

Peel the tangerines and divide into wedges. Set aside. Run through a juicer and transfer to serving glasses.

Stir in the chilled coffee, coconut sugar, and vanilla extract.

Add some ice cubes and serve immediately.

Nutritional information per serving: Kcal: 282, Protein: 6.9g, Carbs: 94g, Fats: 2g

35.   Banana Chokeberry Juice

Ingredients:

1 large banana, peeled

2 cups of chokeberries

2 cups of spinach, torn

2 cups of beet greens, torn

Preparation:

Peel the banana and cut into chunks. Set aside.

Wash the chokeberries under cold running water using a colander. Drain and set aside.

Combine spinach and beet greens in a colander and wash thoroughly. Torn with hands and set aside.

Now, combine banana, berries, spinach, and beet greens in a juicer.

Transfer to serving glasses and add some ice cubes before serving.

Enjoy!

Nutritional information per serving: Kcal: 183, Protein: 7.8g, Carbs: 63.1g, Fats: 1.2g

36.   Pumpkin Cinnamon Juice

Ingredients:

10 oz of pumpkin, chopped

½ tsp of cinnamon, freshly ground

1 cup of sweet potato, chunked

¼ cup of water

Preparation:

Peel the pumpkin and cut in half. Scoop out the seeds and cut into small chunks. Set aside.

Peel the sweet potato and cut into bite-sized pieces. Set aside.

Now, combine pumpkin and sweet potato in a juicer and process until juiced.

Transfer to serving glasses and stir in the water and cinnamon.

Add some ice before serving and enjoy!

Nutritional information per serving: Kcal: 256, Protein: 5.3g, Carbs: 27.8g, Fats: 22.3g

37.   Carrot Apple Juice

Ingredients:

3 large carrots, sliced

2 Granny Smith's apples, cored and chopped

½ tsp of cinnamon, freshly ground

¼ tsp of ginger, ground

1 tbsp of honey, raw

Preparation:

Wash the carrots and chop into thick slices. Set aside.

Wash the apples and remove the core. Cut into bite-sized pieces and set aside.

Combine carrots and apples in a juicer and process until juiced. Transfer to serving glasses and stir in the honey, cinnamon, and ginger.

Add few ice cubes and serve immediately.

Nutritional information per serving: Kcal: 324, Protein: 3.4g, Carbs: 93g, Fats: 1.5g

38.   Grape Vanilla Juice

Ingredients:

1 cup of grapes

1 tsp of pure vanilla extract, sugar-free

2 large bananas, sliced

½ cup of coconut milk, sugar-free

Preparation:

Wash the grapes under cold running water. Drain and set aside.

Peel the bananas and chop into small chunks. Set aside.

Combine bananas and grapes in a juicer and process until juiced. Transfer to serving glasses and stir in the coconut milk and vanilla extract.

Add some ice and serve!

Nutritional information per serving: Kcal: 293, Protein: 7.5g, Carbs: 77.9g, Fats: 4g

39.   Cucumber Grapefruit Juice

Ingredients:

3 large cucumbers, peeled

1 grapefruit, peeled

1 tsp of peppermint extract

1 oz of coconut water

1 tbsp of coconut sugar

Preparation:

Wash the cucumbers and cut into thick slices. Set aside.

Peel the grapefruit and cut into bite-sized pieces. set aside.

Now, combine cucumber and grapefruit in a juicer and process until juiced. Transfer to serving glasses and stir in the coconut water, coconut sugar and peppermint extract.

Add some ice cubes and serve immediately.

Nutritional information per serving: Kcal: 204, Protein: 7.7g, Carbs: 59g, Fats: 1.3g

40.   Flaxseed Banana Juice

Ingredients:

1 tsp of flaxseed oil

1 large banana

1 cup of goji berries

A bunch of celery leaves

1 tbsp of honey, raw

Preparation:

Peel the banana and cut into small chunks. Set aside.

Place the goji berries in a medium bowl and add 1 cup of water. Soak for 30 minutes.

Wash the celery and torn with hands. Set aside.

Now, combine banana, goji berries, and celery in a juicer and process until juiced. Transfer to serving glasses and stir in the flaxseed oil and honey.

Add few ice cubes before serving.

Enjoy!

Nutritional information per serving: Kcal: 177, Protein: 6.5g, Carbs: 44.6g, Fats: 2.6g

41.   Raspberry Cherry Juice

Ingredients:

1 cup of fresh raspberries

½ tsp of pure cherry extract, sugar-free

1 large cucumber, sliced

A couple of mint leaves

Preparation:

Wash the raspberries under cold running water. Drain and set aside.

Wash the cucumber and cut into thin slices. Set aside.

Combine raspberries and cucumber in a juicer and process until juiced. Transfer to serving glasses and stir in the cherry extract.

Garnish with fresh mint leaves and refrigerate for 10 minutes before serving.

Nutritional information per serving: Kcal: 152, Protein: 9.4g, Carbs: 50g, Fats: 2.6g

42.   Blackberry Cucumber Juice

Ingredients:

1 cup of fresh blackberries

1 large cucumber, sliced

1 cup of pomegranate seeds

1 cup of fresh parsley

Preparation:

Wash the blackberries under cold running water. Drain and set aside.

Wash the cucumber and cut into thick slices. Set aside.

Cut the top of the pomegranate fruit using a sharp knife. Slice down to each of the white membranes inside of the fruit. Pop the seeds into a medium bowl.

Wash the parsley thoroughly and roughly chop with hands. Set aside.

Now, combine blackberries, cucumber, pomegranate seeds, and parsley.

Transfer to serving glasses and add some ice cubes before serving.

Nutritional information per serving: Kcal: 143, Protein: 7.9g, Carbs: 44.8g, Fats: 2.5g

43.   Strawberry Ginger Juice

Ingredients:

1 cup of strawberries, fresh

½ tsp of ginger, ground

1 cup of fresh kale, torn

1 whole lemon, peeled

Preparation:

Wash the strawberries under cold running water. Drain and set aside.

Wash the kale thoroughly and torn with hands. Set aside.

Peel the lemon and cut lengthwise in half. Set aside.

Combine strawberries, kale, and lemon in a juicer and process until juiced.

Transfer to serving glasses add some ice cubes before serving.

Enjoy!

Nutritional information per serving: Kcal: 120, Protein: 5.9g, Carbs: 38.6g, Fats: 1.8g

44.   Parsnip Celery Juice

Ingredients:

1 cup of parsnips, chopped

1 celery stalk, chopped

1 whole guava, chopped

2 large grapefruits, peeled

Preparation:

Wash the parsnips and cut into small slices. Set aside.

Wash the celery and cut into small pieces. Set aside.

Wash the guava and cut into chunks. If you are using large fruit, reserve the rest for some other recipe in a refrigerator.

Peel the grapefruits and chop into bite-sized pieces.

Now, combine parsnips, celery, guava, and grapefruits in a juicer and process until juiced.

Transfer to serving glasses and add some ice before serving.

Nutritional information per serving: Kcal: 279, Protein: 7.2g, Carbs: 86g, Fats: 1.7g

45.   Carrot Parsnip Juice

Ingredients:

2 large green apples, peeled and cored

3 large carrots, sliced

1 cup of parsnips, sliced

1 basil leaf, crushed

¼ cup of water

Preparation:

Wash the carrots and parsnips and cut into thick slices. Set aside.

Wash the apples and remove the core. Cut into bite-sized pieces and set aside.

Now, combine carrots, parsnips, and apples in a juicer and process until juiced.

Transfer to serving glasses and stir in the water. Garnish with basil leaves and refrigerate before serving.

Enjoy!

Nutritional information per serving: Kcal: 332, Protein: 5.4g, Carbs: 100g, Fats: 1.6g

46.   Artichoke Lemon Juice

Ingredients:

7 oz of artichokes, chopped

1 medium-sized lemon, peeled

1 whole avocado, chopped

1 cup of red cabbage, torn

1 cup of green cabbage, torn

Preparation:

Trim off the outer leaves of the artichoke using a sharp knife. Cut into small pieces and set aside.

Peel the lemon and cut lengthwise in half. Set aside.

Peel the avocado and cut in half. Remove the pit and cut into chunks. Set aside.

Combine red and green cabbage in a colander and wash under cold running water. Drain and torn with hands. Set aside.

Now, combine artichoke, lemon, avocado, and cabbages in a juicer and process until juiced.

Transfer to serving glasses and add some ice before

serving.

Enjoy!

Nutritional information per serving: Kcal: 353, Protein: 12.3g, Carbs: 51g, Fats: 30g

47.   Cabbage Orange Juice

Ingredients:

1 cup of purple cabbage, torn

1 large orange, peeled

1 cup of papaya, chopped

1 cup of goji berries

1 tsp of ginger, ground

1 tsp of honey

Preparation:

Wash the cabbage thoroughly and torn with hands. Set aside.

Peel the orange and divide into wedges. Set aside.

Peel the papaya and cut lengthwise in half. Scoop out the black seeds and flesh using a spoon. Cut into small chunks and set aside.

Place the goji berries in a bowl and add 1 cup of water. Soak for 30 minutes before juicing.

Combine cabbage, orange, papaya, and goji berries in a juicer and process until juiced.

Transfer to serving glasses and stir in the ginger and honey.

Add some ice cubes and serve immediately.

Nutritional information per serving: Kcal: 172, Protein: 4.3g, Carbs: 54.2g, Fats: 0.7g

ADDITIONAL TITLES FROM THIS AUTHOR

70 Effective Meal Recipes to Prevent and Solve Being Overweight: Burn Fat Fast by Using Proper Dieting and Smart Nutrition

By

Joe Correa CSN

48 Acne Solving Meal Recipes: The Fast and Natural Path to Fixing Your Acne Problems in Less Than 10 Days!

By

Joe Correa CSN

41 Alzheimer's Preventing Meal Recipes: Reduce or Eliminate Your Alzheimer's Condition in 30 Days or Less!

By

Joe Correa CSN

70 Effective Breast Cancer Meal Recipes: Prevent and Fight Breast Cancer with Smart Nutrition and Powerful Foods

By

Joe Correa CSN

www.ingramcontent.com/pod-product-compliance
Lightning Source LLC
Chambersburg PA
CBHW030301030426
42336CB00009B/476